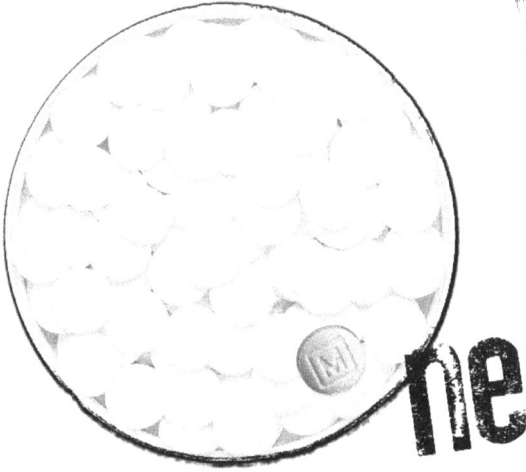

One Pill Killed

Fentanyl Poisoning.
Are you next?

NBI
Normandy's Bright Ideas
Florida

One Pill Killed: Fentanyl Poisoning. Are you Next?
By Normandy D. Piccolo
Printed in the United States of America
Copyright ©2023 by Normandy's Bright Ideas
ISBN: 979-8-9855654-3-0

Credits: Vecteezy, Medic10, NDP, Drug Free, DEA

www.normandydpiccolo.com

TRIGGER WARNING

One Pill Killed discusses the serious and difficult issue of counterfeit medications which are being purchased by users and killing hundreds of people every single day. In fact, every seven minutes, one person dies from an overdose or from being poisoned by a counterfeit drug.

The most common ages of people dying are 18-24 years old. But the ages have been as young as 9 years old and going up to 45 years old and sometimes, even older. Most of those people did not realize they purchased a deadly counterfeit pill. They were poisoned.

They did not overdose.

THEY WERE POISONED.

Per the DEA (Drug Enforcement Administration), some of the most common counterfeit pills on the market that are made to look like prescription opioids are oxycodone (Oxycontin®, Percocet®), hydrocodone (Vicodin®), and alprazolam (Xanax®); or stimulants like amphetamines (Adderall®).

There is also evidence of methamphetamine and marijuana being laced unknowingly with lethal amounts of Fentanyl, resulting in the same deadly consequences as if one were to have swallowed, shot-up, smoked or snorted a counterfeit pill.

Fentanyl is being added to every type of drug.

If you have questions or need assistance, please text The National Helpline at 988 or call the SAMHSA Hotline (Substance Abuse and Mental Health Services) at 1-800-662-4357.

It does not take long to swallow, snort, shoot-up or smoke a counterfeit pill and die.

Based on the amount of Fentanyl that the counterfeit pill has been laced with, it takes less than a few moments for a person to be poisoned.

You stop breathing.

Your brain begins to shrink and suffer irreversible damage.

Your heart stops beating.

And more...

If not treated in time with Narcan, you will die. And even then, with six or eight doses of Narcan trying to reverse the poisonous effects of Fentanyl in your body – it is not enough. You still die.

Off to the morgue you then go.

One last 'ride' you did not plan on experiencing when taking that counterfeit pill.

Is the 'ride' you so desperately seek to experience, worth winding up on a cold, metal table? Dead?

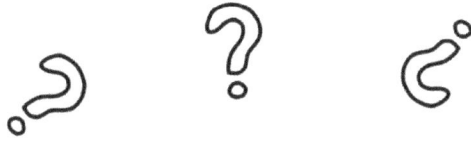

Introduction

One Pill Killed: Fentanyl Poisoning. Are you Next? is to inform you about the dangers of Fentanyl Poisoning. Fentanyl Poisoning is an out of control, growing epidemic few people seem to be aware of that is happening right under their noses.

This book is also designed to make you think twice about taking that pill you bought or were given by a friend. There is a 70% chance (or higher) that pill could be counterfeit. Fake. Pure poison.

Sure, your Plug or Bestie may have assured you that pill is a Perky/Percocet. But is it? Or is it a pill that contains no Percocet or any ingredients included in a real Percocet pill at all.

What if, instead, that pill you are about to take is counterfeit and contains **FIVE TIMES the LETHAL LIMIT** of **FENTANYL.** You will most likely be dead before help arrives.

So, ask yourself, while staring down at that pill in your hand, "Could this pill actually be poison and not what I think it is?"

"Could this be the very last pill I will ever take? Not because I decided to get clean. But because the last pill I took was counterfeit. It was poison and it poisoned me."

Snort it. Shoot it up. Smoke it. Swallow it.

Don't take it.

Ultimately, the decision is yours...

3

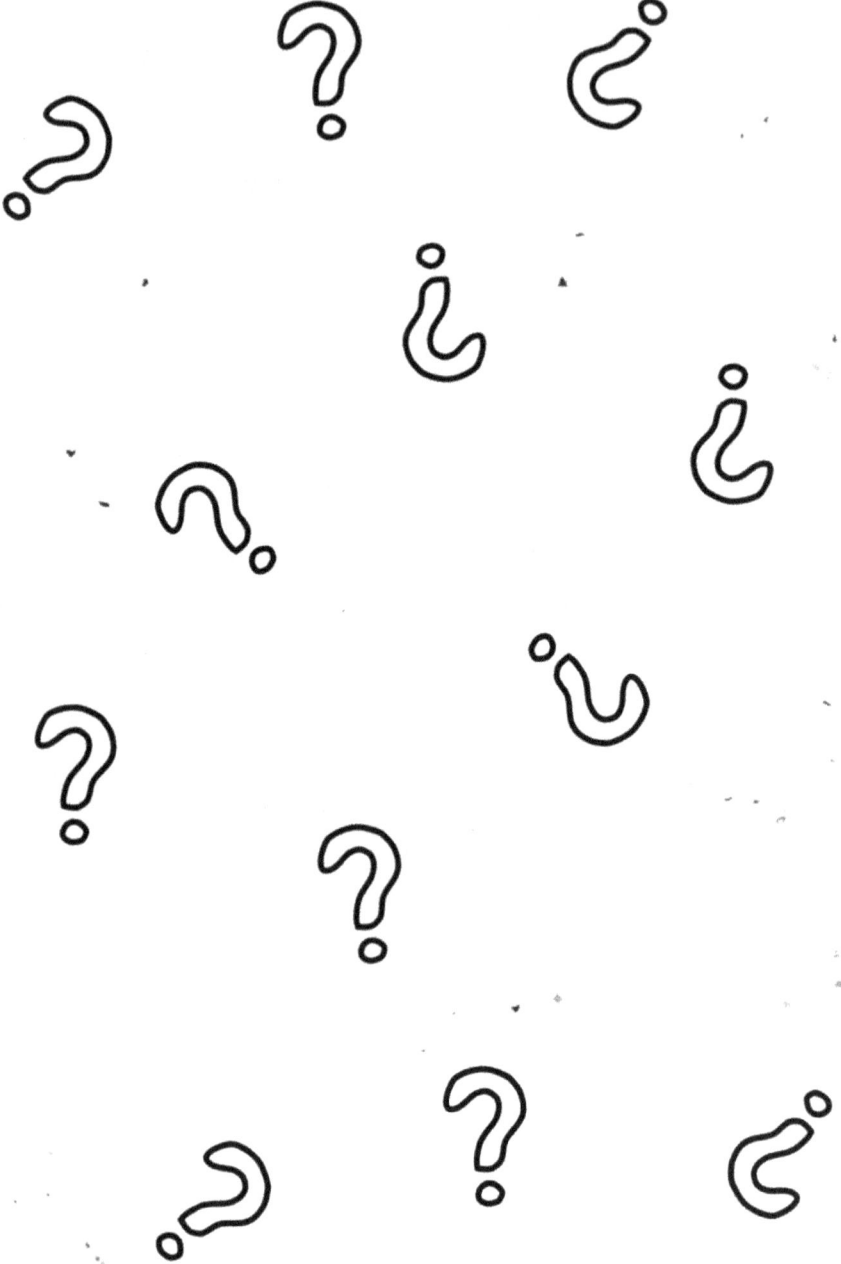

My name **was** Blu...

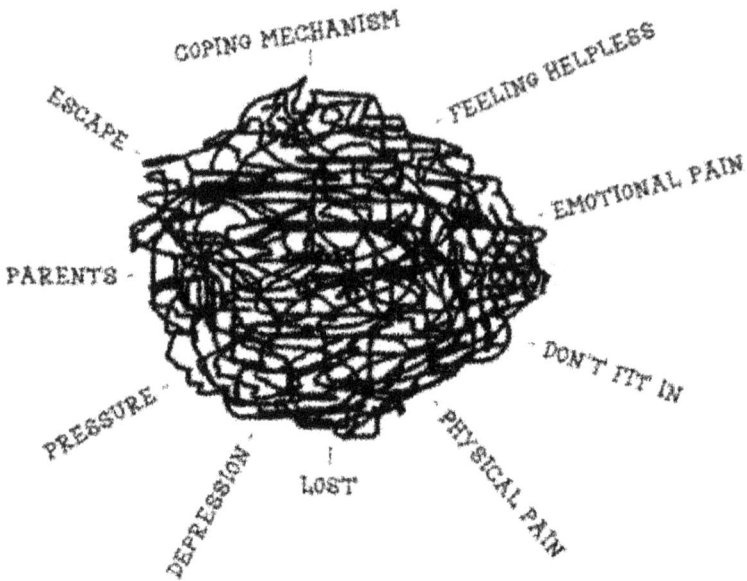

COPING MECHANISM
FEELING HELPLESS
ESCAPE
EMOTIONAL PAIN
PARENTS
DON'T FIT IN
PRESSURE
PHYSICAL PAIN
DEPRESSION
LOST

Up above were some of the many things that once went on inside my brain. Literally 24/7. Sometimes just one. Sometimes more than one. Sometimes it felt like all of them hit me simultaneously.

I hated being me most of the time. But, after being poisoned by a counterfeit M30, now, I would give anything to be chaotic, stressed out, lost, etc....basically me again. But I can't.

My brain, my life felt like utter madness. I sometimes needed an escape. You know, to shut it all down. I knew about M30's. Most people at my school, and even where I worked, knew about them

6

and how to get them, too. Apps. It was as easy as ordering take-out food.

I would swallow an M30 on a bad day and suddenly it felt as if everything went from turmoil to peaceful. Just one pill and BOOM! Life-felt great again. M30's made me be the person I thought I wanted to be instead of the person I was without its powdery wonder dust coursing throughout my body.

I wish I knew then what I know now.

It was all a huge lie. All of it.

The M30's did not change anything negative in my life into a positive. They only made me feel even more destroyed from the inside out. Sure, they made me feel great in the moment - but it was always a short-lived greatness. Whatever I was trying to escape from would always find me again once the pill wore off.

I got lucky for such a long time. I had a reliable Plug. A few close friends whom I could score M30's from anytime I needed one.

Until I took that one pill....and my luck ran out.

There had been rumors and even stories on the news about people being poisoned by taking fake pills. Not overdosing. They were unknowingly getting drugs tainted with Fentanyl. Counterfeits they called them. Sometimes the M30's weren't even M30's. But pure Fentanyl instead. People were being poisoned.

The media talked a lot about the counterfeit M30's and other fake drugs going around tainted with deadly amounts of Fentanyl. I should have listened. But being young, I felt invincible and ignored the warnings.

"It might happen to others, but it will never happen to me. I had a solid Plug and trusted friends who would never do me wrong."

Yet, another lie.

I was feeling depressed one afternoon, so I asked a friend of mine if I could score an M30 from a few she had just bought the night before from a Plug. I trusted her. I planned to take the pill later that night. I was tired of feeling bad and wanted to feel good - even if only for a little while.

Later that night, after my parents had gone to sleep, I fished the pill out of my black purse and swallowed it. I never even bothered to look at the pill before I took it. Why would I? I had gotten it from a friend. A friend who had gotten from a Plug I assumed she knew and trusted, so the pill was a real M30 and safe to take, right? WRONG!

The last thing I remember after swallowing the pill was immediately feeling super sleepy and weak. Then.... nothing. Only permanent darkness. Not even the sounds of my screaming, wailing parents and brother. The paramedics who pushed Narcan up my nose six times and tried everything they could to bring me back failed to wake me up.

My brain had begun to shrink causing irreversible brain damage. My skin went from grey, to blue to purple. My lungs stopped taking in air. My heart no longer beat. My bladder soaked my jeans. I had small chunks of vomit oozing out of my right nostril and mouth. My eyes remained open and rolled back into my head.

I was poisoned by a Fentanyl laced, M30. One counterfeit pill killed me. It can kill you, too. Don't think that it can't happen to you. Because it can. It happened to me, and I never thought it would. But it did.

My dreams.
My aspirations.
My goals.
My hopes.
My future.
My life.
They all disappeared with me.

One poisonous counterfeit pill stole those things from me. Are you going to allow a counterfeit pill to do the same thing to you, too?

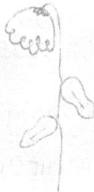

RIP Blu

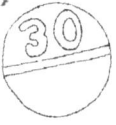

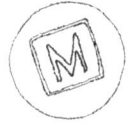

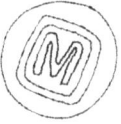

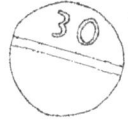

Can you tell the difference?

*Counterfeit pills can be pressed into the identical shape and size as the real pharmaceutical pills they are making thanks in part to skilled pill 'poison' pressers.

*Counterfeit pills come in various colors/shades and can look just like real pharmaceutical pills which Plugs then sell to you. Did you know that six out of ten pills being sold are fake? That is a 70% chance (or higher) of you taking a pill with **FIVE TIMES the LETHAL LIMIT** of **FENTANYL** in it. Is 70% (or higher) worth the risk?

*Can you even tell the difference between the numbers that are stamped on the back of pharmaceutical pills vs a number stamped on a counterfeit pill? Or if the number stamped on the counterfeit pill is a copycat number of the real manufacturers number now designed to trick you into unknowingly taking a fake pill loaded with deadly Fentanyl and not the pill you thought you got? A pill certain to poison you?

If you choose to purchase a pill from a Plug or get it from a friend, are you even sure the pill is what they claim that pill to be? Or could it be a counterfeit pill full of lethal fentanyl, along with other ingredients that will aid in poisoning you to death?

Think before you 'take that ride'. Because you might not be taking the ride you had planned after encountering a counterfeit pill. But rather, you may wind up taking an unplanned ride straight to the County Morgue.

Is taking that ride by encountering a pill you have no idea is real or counterfeit worth the possibility of accidentally ending your life due to being poisoned?

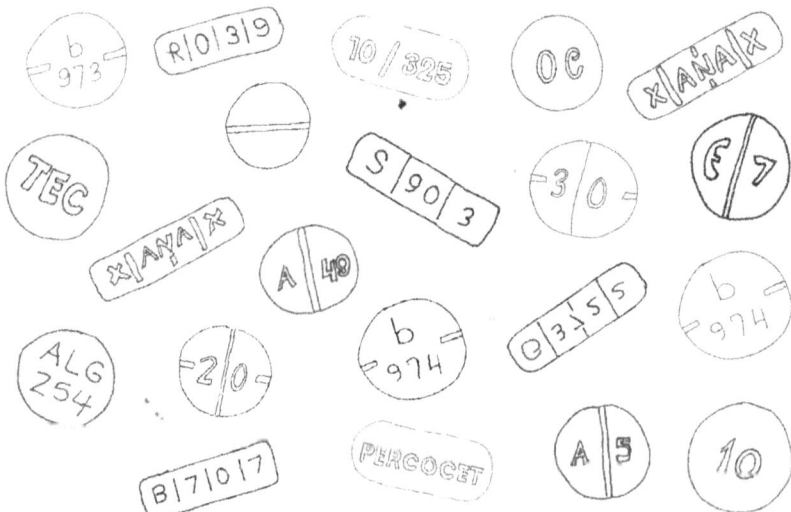

Instagram   TikTok   Snapchat

S CIAL MEDIA

Facebook   X (formally Twitter) & Other Apps...

Social Media sites are a well-known, no-brainer way to connect with a Plug (Drug Dealer) and get any drug your still beating heart desires to take. It's as easy as ordering a spoiled pizza.

It only takes one time for you to end up with a counterfeit pill and flatlining your heart due to unknowingly being poisoned with a lethal dose of Fentanyl.

In other words, take the wrong pill and chances are, no more heartbeat. Ever!

Sure, some people beat the odds and barely get saved from the deadly clutches of Fentanyl Poisoning. But ask yourself this question:

"Is my life worth gambling it on some random pill I purchased from a Plug or got from a friend who most likely got it from a Plug...because chances are if it is a bad pill, I will be saved. I will beat the odds."

Do you honestly believe you can beat five-times the lethal dose of Fentanyl, along with a drug called

13

Carefentanil – a drug made to sedate elephants some dealers are now throwing into the mix? Think about how small you are compared to an elephant. Like an ant easily stomped by an uncaring Plug who most likely, deliberately sold you pure poison.

YOU: Splat! Flatlined! Dead!

PLUG: Richer now thanks to your money.

Big Time Drug Dealers: Keep on making that money as the bodies continually hit the floor - literally.

But being poisoned would never happen to you, right? Better rethink that scenario again before reaching out to a Plug on a social media app or even getting it from a friend who obtained said drug from a Plug they hooked up with.

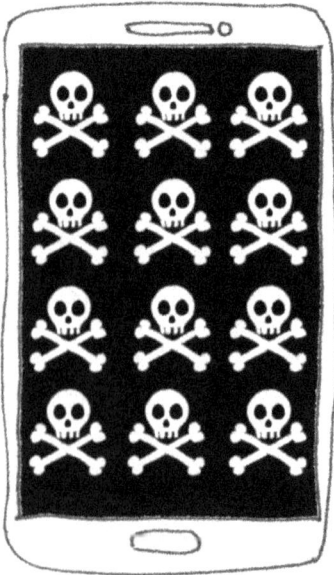

1-800- Plurderer – (A Plug who is a murderer) These Plugs knowingly sell counterfeit drugs laced with lethal Fentanyl to unsuspecting customers and poison them. They have no conscience. Nor do their bosses. It's all about making that money. Your life means nothing to them. But what money they can get from you...that matters.

While buying pills online may appear to be a win-win, it's anything but...at least for you.

You want the high.

The Plug wants your money.

The problem is you are the one taking the risk with your life.

The Plug's only risk is some jail time if caught.

But the Plug gets to live on and eventually returns to dealing deadly, counterfeit, poisonous pills again.

While you on the other hand get to do nothing.

Because you, my friend, are done. Dead. Dusted.

You unknowingly took a pill laced with Fentanyl.

You were poisoned. Your life is over.

PILL ROULETTE

PILL ROULETTE

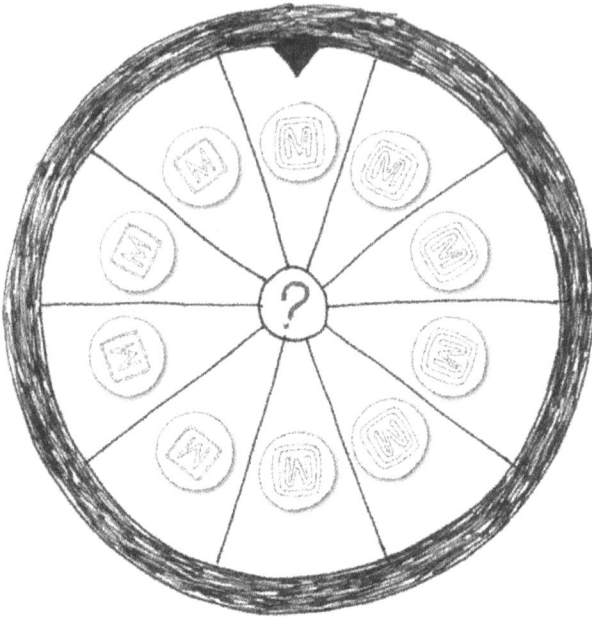

Before you spin the wheel of 'Pill Roulette' above, certain you are going to win and land a real pill and not a counterfeit that could poison you to death with Fentanyl, you should know:

In 2022, FOUR out of TEN pills were found to be laced with lethal amounts of Fentanyl.

In 2023, SEVEN out of TEN pills were found to be laced with lethal amounts of Fentanyl.

That is a guaranteed 70% chance (or higher) you will encounter a deadly pill that will poison you. And the odds of that lethal encounter keep climbing.

So…do you like those odds? You know, the House always wins in the end, right?

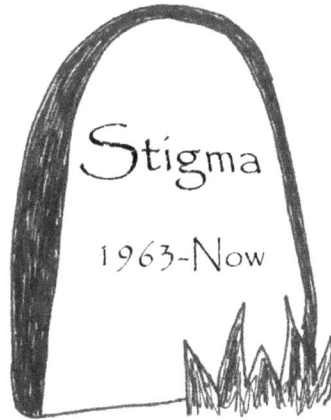

Stigma
1963-Now

The time of death – the day of DEATH for
STIGMA is RIGHT NOW!

No more Stigma regarding Fentanyl Poisoning, accidental overdosing, or drug addiction in general.

Or having Narcan on hand in case of an overdose.

Don't you think it's time to stop caring what others might think of you, your loved one, etc....?

What is more important?

Their life or Your pride?

You decide...

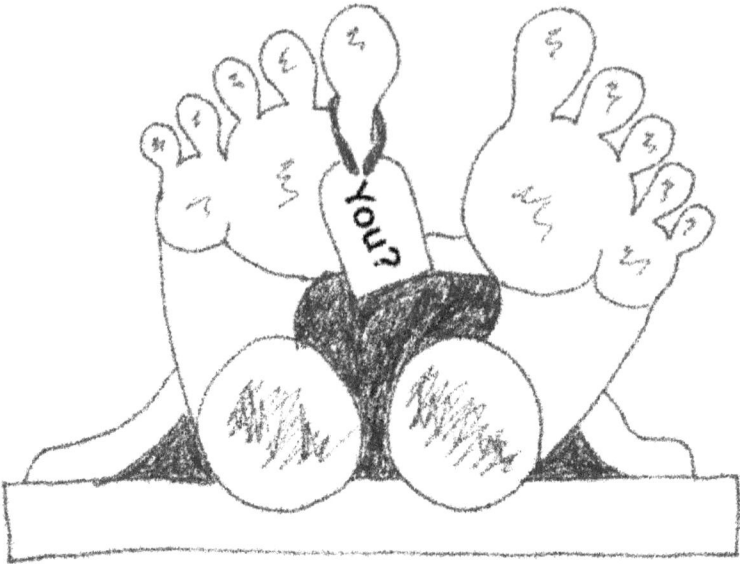

YOUR LIFE is not a game when it comes to getting drugs from the streets or via Social Media Apps... though you might think otherwise.

So, the question remains....

TAG!

Are you it?

The Ripple Effect

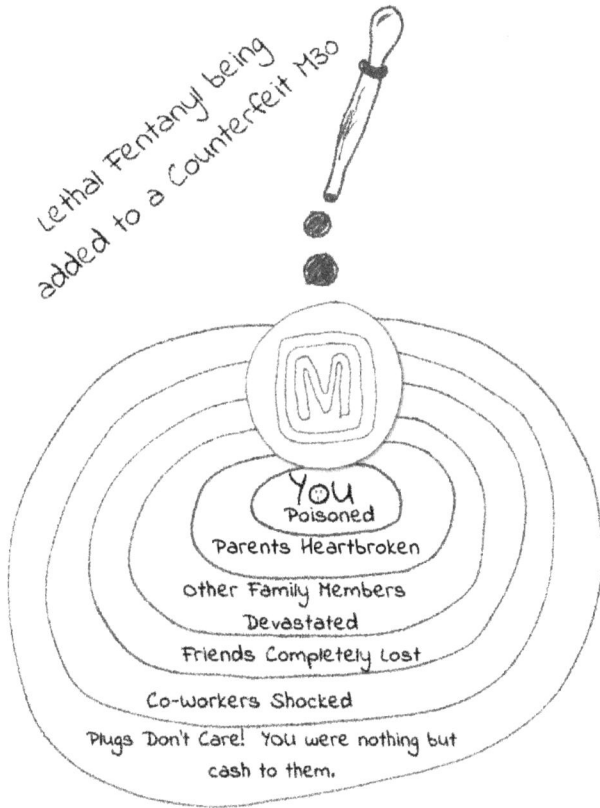

Lethal Fentanyl being added to a Counterfeit M30

YOU
Poisoned

Parents Heartbroken

Other Family Members Devastated

Friends Completely Lost

Co-workers Shocked

Plugs Don't Care! You were nothing but cash to them.

Being poisoned by Fentanyl via a counterfeit pill doesn't just affect you. It affects everyone in your life...except for Plugs. You were nothing but a cash cow to a Plug. You will be replaced by another customer, who will unknowingly be poisoned just like you were, before the coroner even arrives on scene to collect your cold. dead body. That is how little dealers care about poisoning you. It's all about making money for them. Nothing more. Get it?

Flexin' Those Zeros

Oh, I'm not talking about showing off how much money a Plug makes from customers they have sold their poisonous garbage too.

Plugs are known to make a lot of money. But they are not the only ones making money off your life when selling you something spiked with **FIVE TIMES** the **LETHAL LIMIT of FENTANYL.**

In the drug business, the money trickles upward, not downward. Even more Zeros/losers who are poisoning you to save them money.

Plugs love to flex on the web about how much money they made off unfortunate 'marks' like you- along with pictures of whatever other poisonous, counterfeit junk they are currently peddling.

Long gone are the days of being screwed over by a dealer who sold you a Vitamin pill instead of the drug you wanted. Back then, you got a harmless vitamin that would do nothing to you. No high. No death. You were just out a few bucks. And rightly pissed off. But you were still alive. Not anymore.

Think about it for a minute. Plugs might be flexin' those zeros from cash made off people they murdered by knowingly, (though some claim they did not know), selling customers poisonous junk. Dealers have you thinking not only are they heroes earning all those zeros from people like you looking for a high, but they're so cool and honest.

LIES! All of it! Remember earlier – **70% (or higher)** of drugs being sold now are counterfeit and laced with deadly amounts of Fentanyl. Your odds are very high of encountering a deadly drug. Is it starting to sink in, yet?

The only true Zeros being flexed on the streets or Internet Apps are the Plugs themselves. They are 100% losers. And so, too, is anyone involved in making these poisonous pills and putting them on the streets or Internet Apps.

Because only a loser and their "business associates", and very sick ones at that, would deliberately sell lethal Fentanyl laced products to unknowing customers and poison those customers TO DEATH in order to save a buck on the dealer's end. Because believe it or not, losing customers is no biggie. There are always more customers willing to take the gamble. Customers – You- while not replaceable to your family, are replaceable to a drug dealer.

Each one of those "ZEROS" flexed by a Plug on the web most likely represents someone's life who was taken due to being poisoned by Fentanyl.

OOOOOOOOOOOOOOOOOOOOOOOOOOOOOOOOOOOOOOOOOOOOO
OOOOOOOOOOOOOOOOOOOOOOOOOOOOOOOOOOOOOOOOOOOOO
OOOOOOOOOOOOOOOOOOOOOOOOOOOOOOOOOOOOOOOOOOOOO
OOOOOOOOOOOOOOOOOOOOOOOOOOOOOOOOOOOOOOOOOOOOO
OOOOOOOOOOOOOOOOOOOOOOOOOOOOOOOOOOOOOOOOOOOOO
OOOOOOOOOOOOOOOOOOOOOOOOOOOOOOOOOOOOOOOOOOOOO
OOOOOOOOOOOOOOOOOOOOOOOOOOOOOOOOOOOOOOOOOOOOO
OOOOOOOOOOOOOOOOOOOOOOOOOOOOOOOOOOOOOOOOOOOOO
OOOOOOOOOOOOOOOOOOOOOOOOOOOOOOOOOOOOOOOOOOOOO
OOOOOOOOOOOOOOOOOOOOOOOOOOOOOOOOOOOOOOOOOOOOO
OOOOOOOOOOOOOOOOOOOOOOOOOOOOOOOOOOOOOOOOOOOOO
OOOOOOOOOOOOOOOOOOOOOOOOOOOOOOOOOOOOOOOOetc…

A SHOCKING DEAL

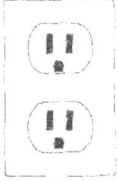

You got any M30's?

How many?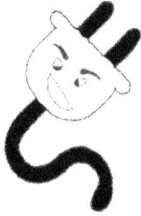

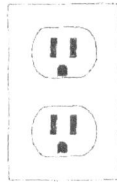 one.

Customer pays the Plug for what they think is an actual M30. Plug delivers a counterfeit M30 pill to the customer instead. Customer took the unknowing counterfeit M30 and got fried. The customer allowed the wrong dealer to "plug in".

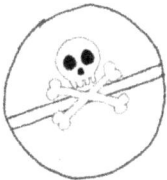

Counterfeit M30

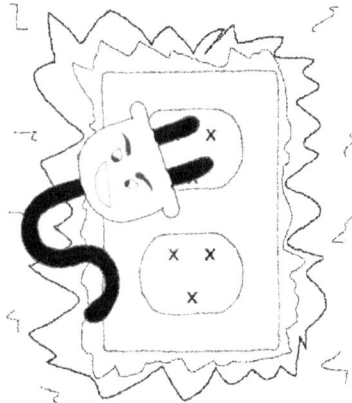

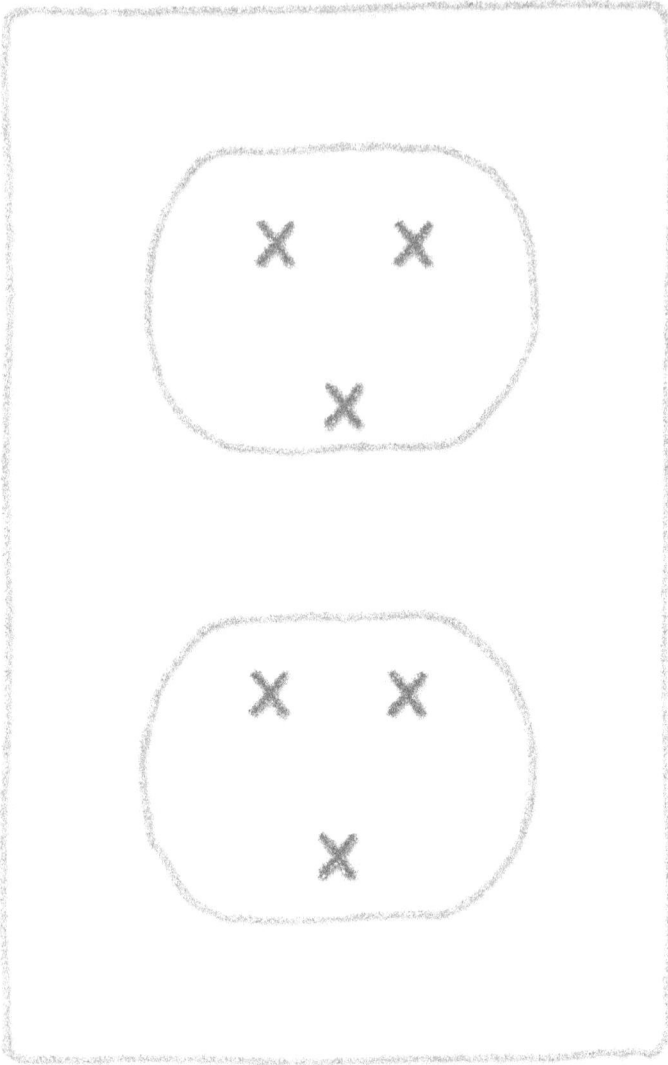

Gone Too Soon...

"I ordered an Adderall and got a Franken-Pill instead. WTF?"

This is only some of the harmful and possibly deadly ingredients found in Counterfeit "Franken-Pills".

So, what is a Franken-Pill? Turn the page and find out....

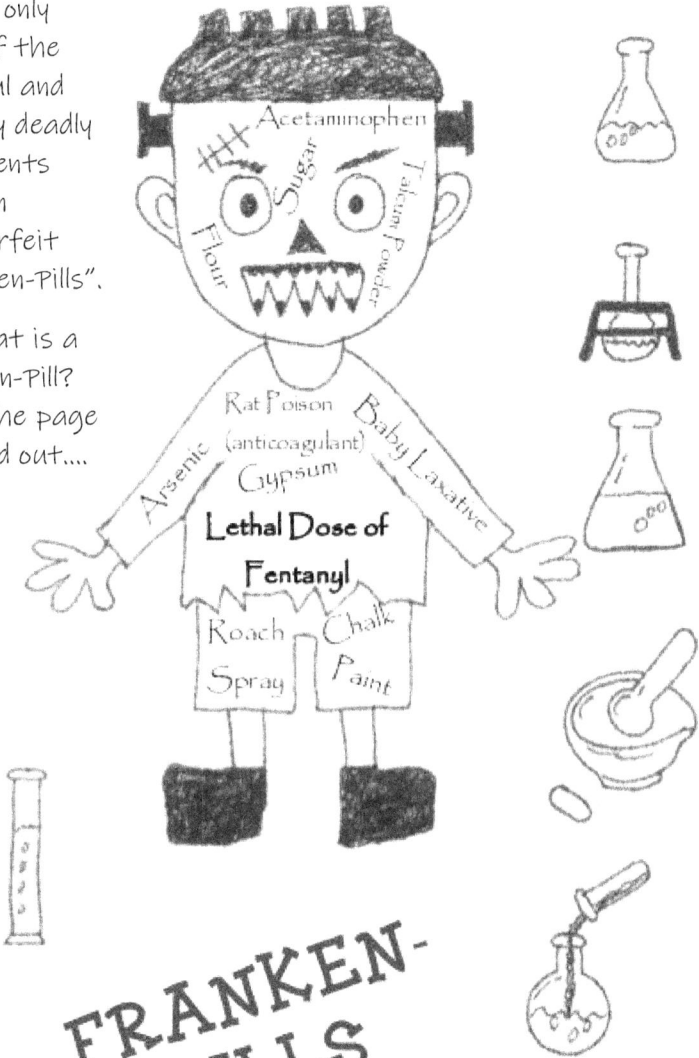

Acetaminophen
Sugar
Talcum Powder
Flour

Rat Poison (anticoagulant)
Arsenic
Baby Laxative
Gypsum

Lethal Dose of Fentanyl

Koach Spray
Chalk Paint

FRANKEN-PILLS

Notice how in the Franken-Pill drawing, there is not one ingredient for a real Adderall/Addy Pill listed? A true Adderall Pill, contains the following:

ACTIVE INGREDIENTS:
dextroamphetamine saccharate, amphetamine aspartate, dextroamphetamine sulfate and amphetamine sulfate.

INACTIVE INGREDIENTS:
colloidal silicon dioxide,
compressible sugar,
corn starch,
magnesium stearate,
microcrystalline cellulose
and saccharin sodium.

All ingredients shown on the Franken-Pill diagram on page 25 show nothing but mostly ingredients that will poison you - except for two (if taken in small quantities). The baby laxative and acetaminophen.

There was not one true Adderall ingredient added to that 'alleged' Adderall Pill a customer purchased in good faith. It was never an Adderall pill. Only the customer was unaware that what they had purchased was a 100% Lethal counterfeit pill.

Date of their Death: Last night.

Why are you deliberately choosing to take a **70% chance (or higher)** risk of encountering a counterfeit pill all in the hopes of a temporary escape from whatever issues you are dealing with?

There must be a better way.
There is a better way.
A safer way.
A healthier way.

You need to deal with your issues and then you will heal. Running away or masking any past hurts or problems with substances never works. The 'High' always wears off and eventually brings you back to the 'Low'.

Aren't you tired of being low?

Are you aware that Franken-Pills (aka: Lethal Counterfeit Fentanyl laced Pills) are made in dirty, nasty, filthy, disgusting, unsanitary labs in Mexico before being distributed to the public? The ingredients for making Fentanyl come from China and India. Easier and scarier to order than you might realize. Selling those ingredients is big business, especially over in China.

You are lucky if the 'chemist-flunkies', playing mad scientist, making your lethal counterfeit pills wash their hands after taking a pee before continuing onward before a pill presser takes over and completes the job.

Did you also know that the Dr. Franken-Pill wannabes who are making the lethal counterfeit pills have no idea what they are doing? No real recipe which they follow when whipping up these batches of deadly 'Betty Croaker" ready to hit the streets and internet and poison you?

Think about it....

How do you suppose it always works out where one batch of drugs hits the streets that are not as deadly. Yeah, some people overdose or get poisoned, but not a large amount by their (dealers) standards.

But then suddenly the next batch to hit the streets literally kills anyone who takes it? Now how do you suppose that happens? Brainless 'Betty Croaker's' doing the cooking and cheap Drug Lords trying to spread out their supply and save themselves money - that's how.

Try and picture a bunch of uneducated, baker-wannabe, low-paid workers that are crammed into disgusting bathrooms - probably crawling with cockroaches. or in filthy factories, and who knows what other type of unsanitary buildings, basically winging-it and making deadly counterfeit pills especially for you.

These 'Betty Croakers' probably never even bother to clean their cooking supplies after making each batch. Nasty! And thus, upping the odds of making the next batch they cook even more deadly than the batch before it.

Ashes to ashes.
Dust to dust.
Take that lethal, Fentanyl-laced
counterfeit pill.
And end up with a **70% chance (or higher)**
of being killed.

Truth be told, most 'Betty Croakers' are working like underpaid dogs. They are also likely dropping dead like flies on the very tables they are making the drugs on that the Plug will be selling to you on the streets or on an App to swallow, smoke, shoot-up, or crush and snort. And like you, the dead 'Betty Croaker' is replaced immediately with another.

It is possible some of those 'Betty Croakers' die from using the product themselves. Or because Fentanyl is so deadly, (just two tiny grains the size of salt can kill you), they die via good old-fashioned exposure.

All this death and destruction just so Big-time Dealers can live 'the good life' at so many other people's expense. But everyone underneath them; the workers to the buyers keep them in business. So, you buy drugs from the streets or an App, and you are part of the problem. You are funding and supporting their murderous lifestyle.

Know that the big shots will always cut as many corners as they can when making/selling product, not caring how many coroners have to handle their now ex-customers after said ex-customers overdosed or were poisoned via their knowingly peddled poisonous product.

All anyone in the drug game cares about is a quick turnover to make those zeros... err... I mean become BIGGER ZEROS.

They do not care about you.

You are as replaceable as the money you paid them to die.

So, do you want to keep helping these ZEROS live in the lap of luxury at your expense? Your Life? Your finances? And risk a get high or possibly die scenario on your end?

You decide....

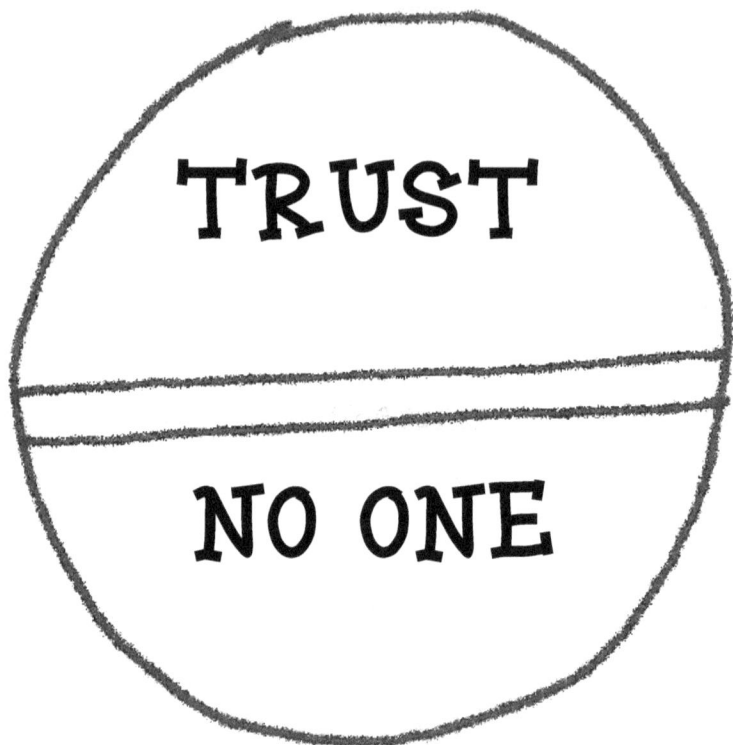

TRUST

NO ONE

Friends or

Plugs.

Consider everyone you get drugs from suspicious. In case you have not figured it out by now, Friends and Plugs can be as fake and counterfeit as the products they are selling or giving to you.

No matter how long these people have been your "homey, reliable, your boo or ride or die" or whatever else you want to label them – all in the name of loyalty. Trust no one.

Stop believing the false pretense Plugs or Friends would ever knowingly screw you over. It can and does happen! More than most realize.

In some cases, it really is an accident and perhaps the Plug or your Friend did not know the drug they sold you or gave to you was a deadly counterfeit. But again, let's repeat those odds of encountering a DEADLY COUNTERFEIT PILL nowadays. Not just a counterfeit pill. But a DEADLY ONE.

70% Chance (or higher) You Will Get Sold or Given a Lethal, Counterfeit Pill. 70% (or higher) CHANCE!

And the odds continue to increase with time. Why? Better profit margins for the Big Time Dealers by creating a cheaper supply using deadly ingredients to make the more expensive ones last longer and go further - thus helping them earn more money by selling lethal pills.

On a side note: They bring continual business to Funeral Homes. (PS: Funeral Homes are not in on it.) But drug dealers sure do keep them in business.

You have no idea where the ingredients or where that drug you got in your hand right now truly came from. China? Mexico? India? You have no idea which 'Betty

Croaker' made it. You have no idea if it is counterfeit. You have no idea if it will kill you instantly or slowly or maybe not at all.... this time. But the odds are (one more time so it really sinks in) it is more than **70% (or higher)** you will purchase or be given a deadly counterfeit pill laced with Five-times the lethal dose of Fentanyl.

Think before you take it. *"Is that pill, that escape, that feel good party moment I'm seeking worth losing my life over?"*

You decide...

Chasing the Dragon

You: "I'm going to get you, Dragon."

Dragon: "No. It is I who is going to get you... in the end."

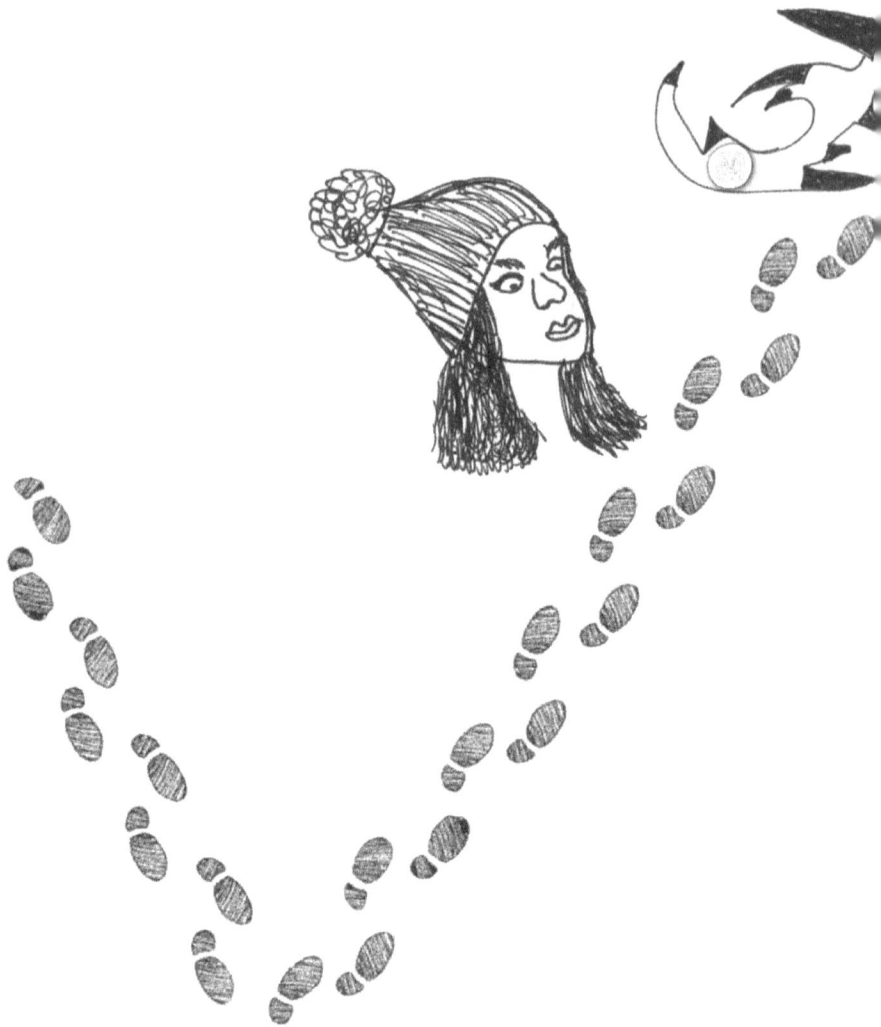

Chasing the Dragon is all about seeking to feel that Super High you felt the first time you took a drug...only you will NEVER FEEL a rush like that again no matter how many drugs you take.

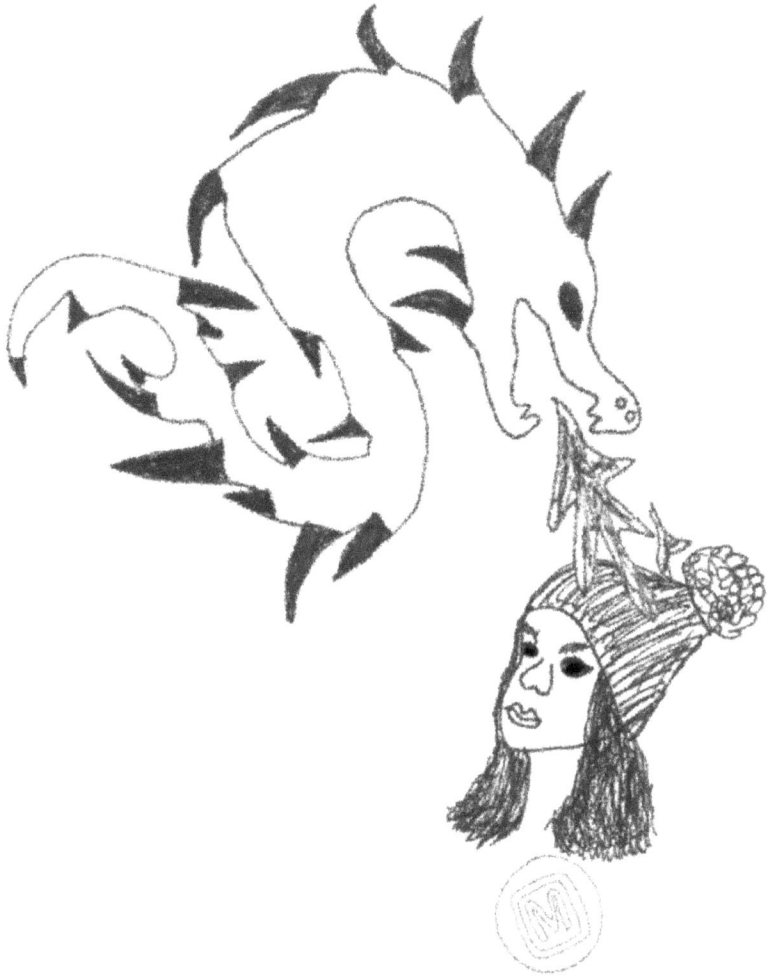

- Chase the Dragon long enough and sooner or later the Dragon will turn around and catch you, burning you into a pile of ashes with its fiery, unforgiving wrath in the form of an overdose or from being unknowingly poisoned.

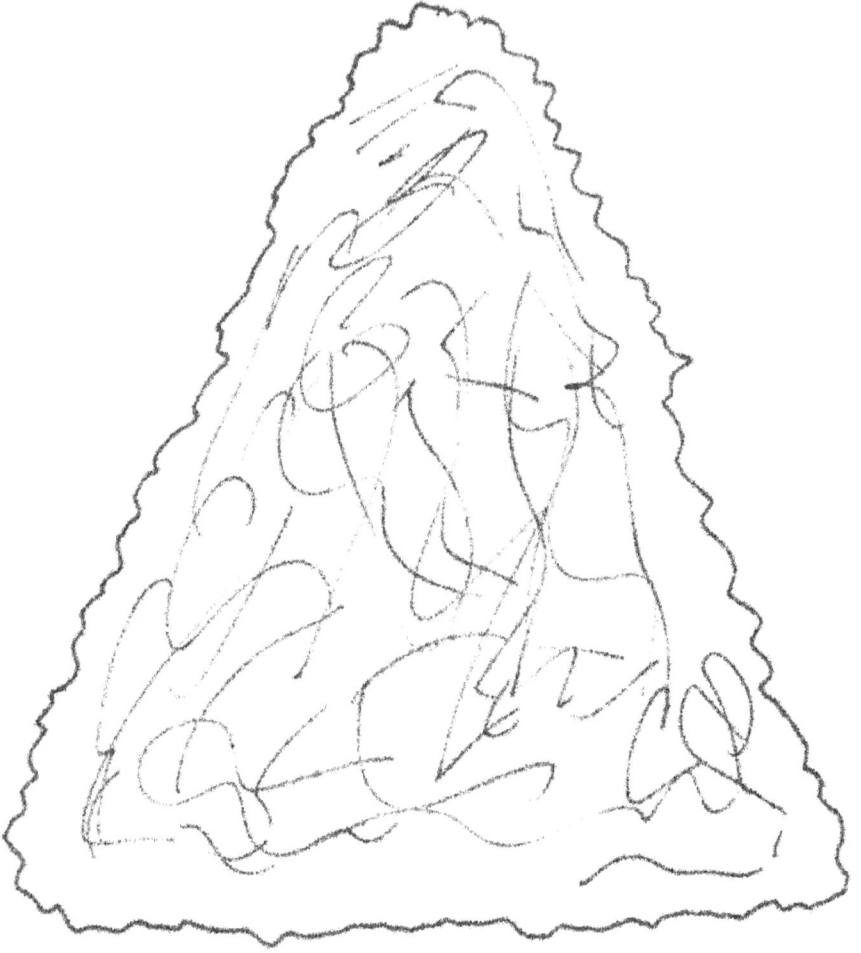

Now, you are nothing but a pile of ashes.

The chase is over and so, too, are you.

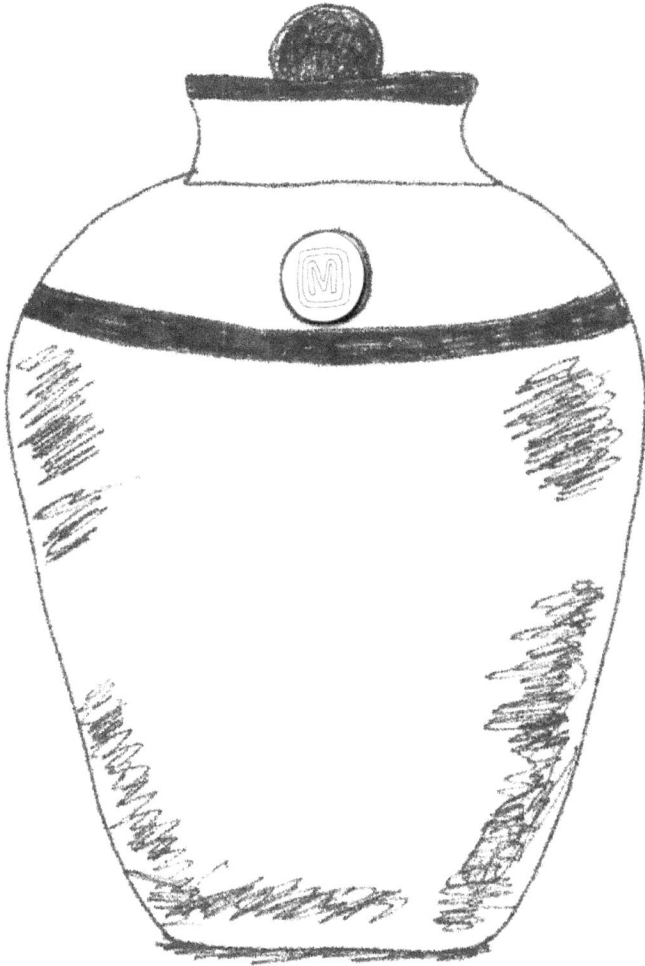

That will be you in that urn if you continue to 'Chase the Dragon'. Snug as a pile of gray ashes crammed into an urn. All that your family has left of you. A pile of ashes. No hopes or dreams for your future. Just your ashes.

To a Dragon Chaser, every day feels like this is going to be that first day, that first time all over again. Only it never is. And it never will be.

It is all a deception in your brain.

Your brain craves that 'feel good' sensation you felt the first time you got high.

From then on, your brain continues to trick you into believing that getting high will bring that same first-time high feeling again. Only it never does.

Your brain also fools you into believing that getting high will solve your problems. But it won't. Pills don't solve problems or heal pain. Like a bad speaker at a concert, pills only serve to make loud, screeching, painful sounds. You never heal. You never deal... well, except when buying drugs.

Making the decision to face your problems and pain and deciding it is time to heal is what solves and heals the pain.

Making the decision to take a counterfeit pill laced with deadly Fentanyl will only get you poisoned - and now your problems have only just begun.

Do not think because you are dead, your troubles are over. They follow you all the way to the grave and haunt you for eternity.

Don't you think it's time to get 'High' on a new thing? Like drug-free things in life.

Maybe even heal from past hurts instead of taking more than a 70% (or higher) chance risk of dying just to escape a bad time in your life by ingesting, smoking, snorting, or shooting up a counterfeit pill?

Your life - you have more value and are more valuable than you realize.

And that my friend, is not a counterfeit statement.

That is a REAL FACT.

BE A
DRAGON SLAYER

Help an addict survive a poisonous overdose.

If you are a user of Opioids, it is very important and wise to always have Narcan available. Narcan can reverse the effects of an opioid overdose. You do not have to be an addict to carry Narcan with you. But you can have it with you just in case. Because you never know when you might be put in a position and encounter someone who is overdosing, and that person needs a Dragon Slayer to try and help save their life. You!

Keep in mind that hospitals and even paramedics working out in the field are encountering counterfeit overdoses in mass quantities. In some states it has gotten so bad, they have had to set up their own "Overdose Squads" that only respond to overdose calls.

Not only are the overdoses themselves massive in the number of people... but it is not like the old days where one or two shots of Narcan up the nostril would bring an overdosing person back from the grip of death.

Nowadays, the lethal amounts of Fentanyl and even sometimes, the drug Carfentanil being added to counterfeit drugs, is so potent that six or even eight doses of Narcan are being used to try and save someone's life. And even that is not enough. The person still dies.

By having Narcan available, you can be one who **'slays the dragon'** addicts or even a one-time user chased that led them into getting burned (poisoned) and help put the metaphoric fire out before they become a pile of ashes in an Urn.

You can be a **'Dragon Slayer'**. A person who helps someone overdosing on an opioid by using Narcan. Narcan is available on-line, at Fire Stations, and Pharmacies. Many times, it is given for free.

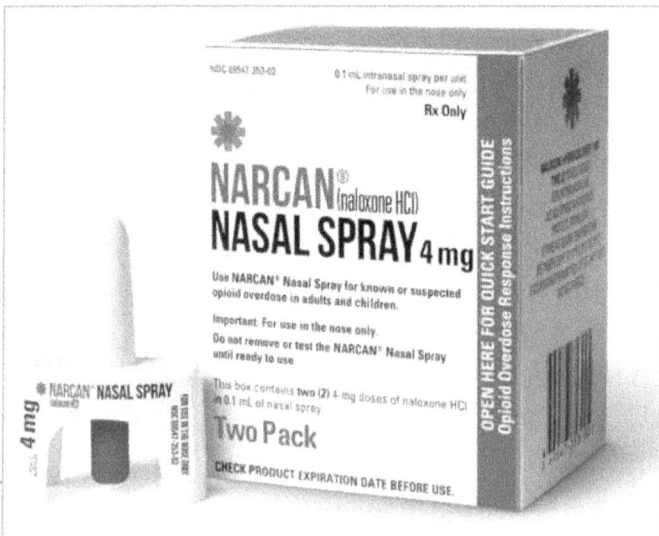

Signs Someone is Overdosing

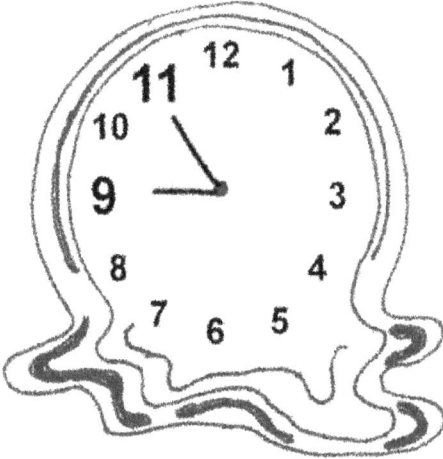

When someone is overdosing, time is of the essence. Every second literally counts in determining their chances of survival. Immediately call 911:

1. Their face is very pale, and they feel clammy to the touch
2. Their body goes limp
3. Pinpoint pupils – the eyes do not respond to changes in light
4. Fingernails and lips turn blue or purple

5. They begin to vomit or make strange gurgling type noises, sometimes like a loud unusual sounding snore
6. You cannot wake them up
7. They cannot speak
8. Their breathing is shallow or not at all
9. Their heart stops beating/no pulse

If the person is not breathing, begin CPR until help arrives. And if you have Narcan on hand, administer it immediately.

Be sure that if the person overdosing begins to respond to the Narcan and starts to come around, gently roll them on their side so they do not choke on their vomit.

FINAL THOUGHTS

Consider getting High on Life in a drug-free way, instead of playing Pill Roulette. The odds are no longer worth it. And they are only going to continue to climb in a direction which is not in your favor.

There are so many things in the world that can help you forget your troubles for the same amount of time as a pill. Healthy things that can give you that amazing endorphin rush you seek to feel so badly from drugs. Only better. And safer.

Exercise, play sports, form a relationship with God (not organized religion), reading, painting, gardening, learn a new language, go back to school, change your life, change your friends. Moving to a new city. Go on an adventure. Do something you have always wanted to do but could not because you were too high on drugs all the time. The list of positive things to do goes on.

Decide what makes you happy.

If you say, *"Taking drugs makes me happy,"* you are not only full of crap, but you are also fooling and lying to yourself.

Taking drugs makes no one happy. It merely masks the pain or whatever issue going on. It will eventually no longer work.

And with dealers being as dirty as they are, it is just a matter of time before one of those, LETHAL COUNTERFEIT PILLS, makes its way into your body via snorting, smoking, shooting-up or being swallowed and killing you - if you choose to remain on your current road.

Newsflash: It's a DEAD-END Road. Literally.

Again, **70% (or higher)** chance the drugs currently being sold on the streets or on Internet Apps are counterfeit and laced with **FIVE TIMES the LETHAL LIMIT of FENTANYL.** And the percentages will only continue to rise as time goes on. This fact cannot be repeated enough.

If you need medication for legitimate medical issues, forget the stigma regarding the medical issue and about what others might think of you and get what you need the safe way. Through a legal prescription. Not from the streets or via a Plug on an App.

But as always, the power always has and always will literally lie in your hands.

Take a good hard look at that potentially deadly counterfeit pill you might be holding in your hand right now and are about to take because you had a bad day, can't cope, feel depressed…basically any excuse will do to feel better and not like crap.

Really look at that pill.

Then stop and think for yourself.

Because ultimately you decide if taking that drug is worth the risk.

One last WARNING: The odds are highly stacked in the negative realm and therefore there is a 70% (or higher) chance they will not fall in your favor. You will most likely be poisoned. You will most likely die.

Is it worth the risk?

You have the power to change your life. You can be counterfeit like the pills by not dealing with your issues. Or you can be real and tell someone how you are feeling and get legit help and legit medication that is safe.

You can choose to manage difficult stuff in life when it happens in a safer, more constructive way and avoid dying, by being poisoned from taking a counterfeit pill.

Remember, if you get lucky and don't take a counterfeit pill – that 'false high' you feel is only temporary. Eventually the pill will wear off and you will feel 'low' again. Continue the cycle and eventually it is a matter of time before you encounter a deadly pill laced with lethal Fentanyl that no amount of Narcan will be able to bring you back from.

I believe in you.

Now believe in yourself.

I hope you make the right choice.

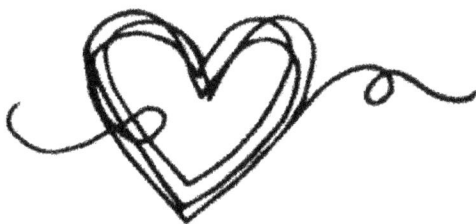

GET HIGH ON A NEW THING... LIFE!

Book Summary

One Pill Killed: Fentanyl Poisoning. Are you Next? is a book/pamphlet to inform you about the dangers of Fentanyl Poisoning. It pulls no punches and is unlike any other book currently on the shelves. You get the facts in a unique, honest way and then you decide what to do with the information.

Fentanyl Poisoning is an out of control, growing epidemic few people seem to be aware of that is happening right under their noses. And it is getting worse by the day.

One Pill Killed: Fentanyl Poisoning. Are you Next? is designed to make you think twice about taking that pill you bought from a Plug or were given to by a friend. Because there is a **70% CHANCE (or HIGHER)** that pill is counterfeit. Fake. It could have **FIVE TIMES THE LETHAL LIMIT OF FENTANYL.**

While staring down at that counterfeit pill in your hand you just bought, ask yourself this question, *"Could this pill actually be poison and not what I think it is and I could die within minutes of taking it?"*

Snort it.
Shoot it up.
Smoke it.
Swallow it.

Don't take it.

Ultimately, the decision is yours...

www.ingramcontent.com/pod-product-compliance
Lightning Source LLC
Chambersburg PA
CBHW060258030426
42335CB00014B/1765